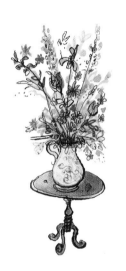

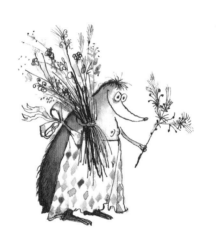

LES TRÈS RICHES HEURES DE MRS MOLE

16th June 1967

16th June 1975

the Beautiful Dream — come true xxx

LES TRÈS RICHES HEURES DE MRS MOLE

Forty-seven drawings made for his wife, Monica, each time she underwent chemotherapy

RONALD SEARLE

blue door

For Monica a.k.a. 'Mrs Mole' who disappeared before she could see her book realised.

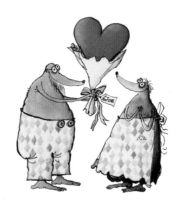

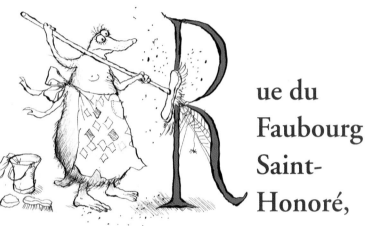

Rue du Faubourg Saint-Honoré, Paris, New Year's Eve, 1969.

Snow in the air, the clatter of shop shutters closing down for the holiday; well-wrapped last-minute shoppers hurrying home with their cagettes of oysters and packets of boudin noir; slightly flushed girls, giggling as they descended the stairs from office parties. All slightly Dickensian. But, for us: DRAMA.

Monica, up in the second-floor doctor's surgery opposite the Elysée Palace, was being diagnosed with a rare, virulent, fatal form of breast cancer. After that, a panic rush to the mammography clinic before it closed. Confirmation: positive. Then, in a state of bewilderment, a taxi home to blow up balloons for our New Year's party that could not be cancelled.

Five years followed of surgery, radiation, medication, scanners, chemotherapy and for me, the intolerable situation of being a helpless bystander, trying to find any possible way of being a support. I thrashed about, desperately seeking whatever small contribution I could make to relieve the pain and suffering. I have only my talent for drawing, so I drew . . .

What emerged was a minuscule, romantic saga of a 'Mrs Mole' pottering about a dream house in a provençal village. This was eventually to be our home, once it had been transformed from its original chaos.

In each of those little private messages, 'Mrs Mole' was present to cheer every dreaded chemotherapy session and evoke the blissful future ahead. Monica had been given six months to live. That was over forty years ago. She beat the unexpected and the seemingly inevitable and now this, miraculously, is her book.

[1]

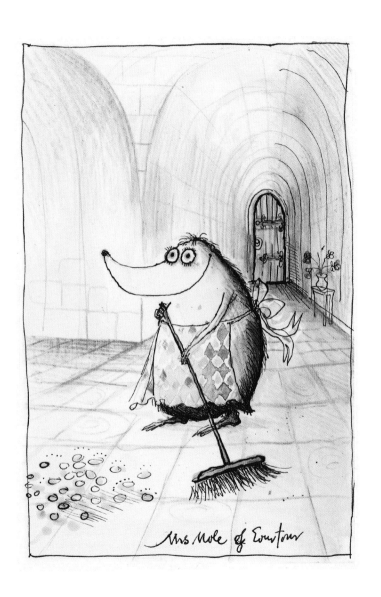

Mrs Mole of Courtour

[2]

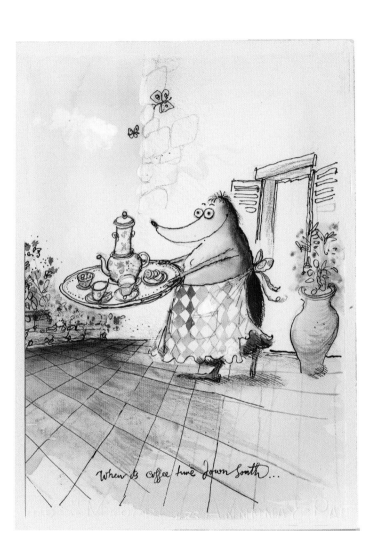

When it's coffee time down South...

[3]

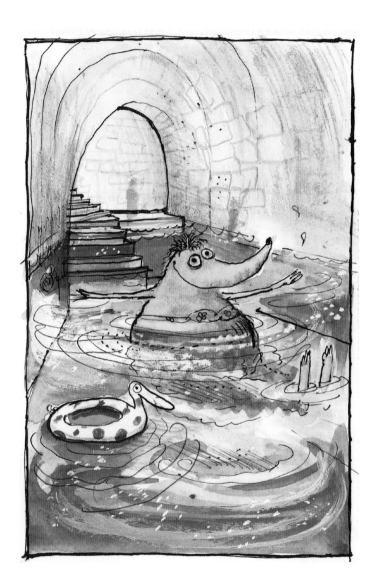

[4]

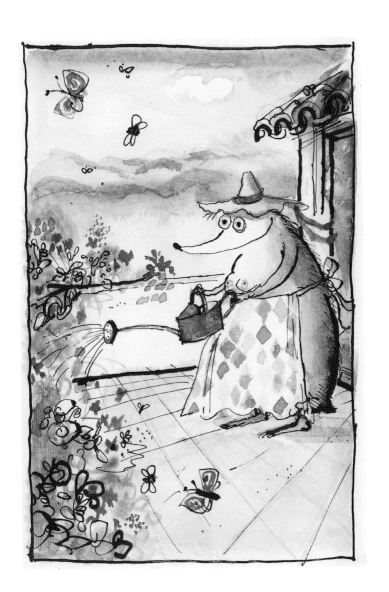

[5]

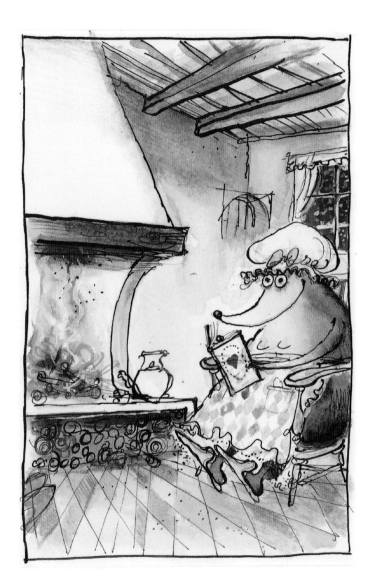

[6]

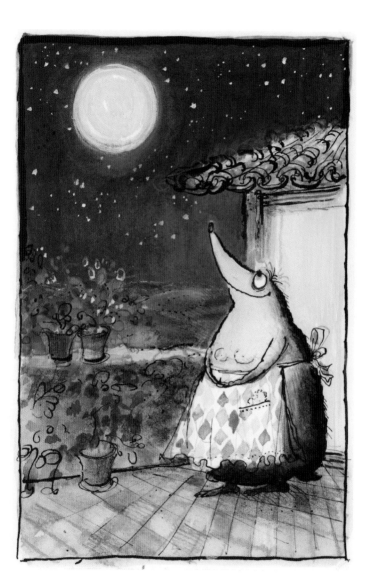

[7]

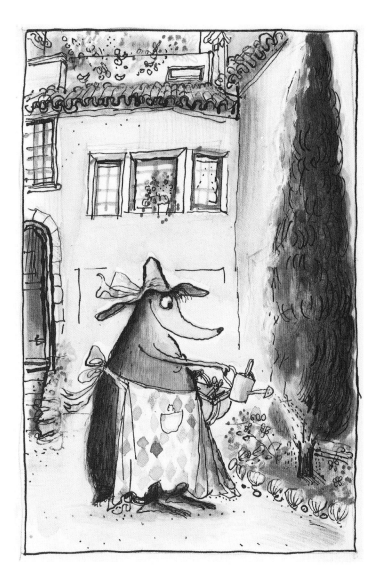

[8]

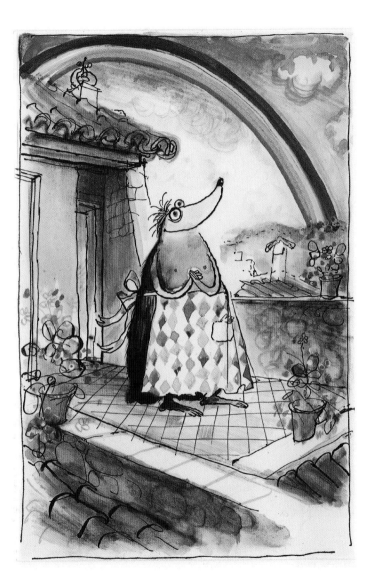

[9]

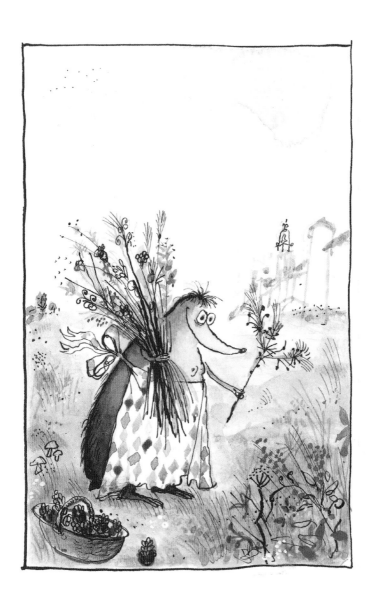

[10]

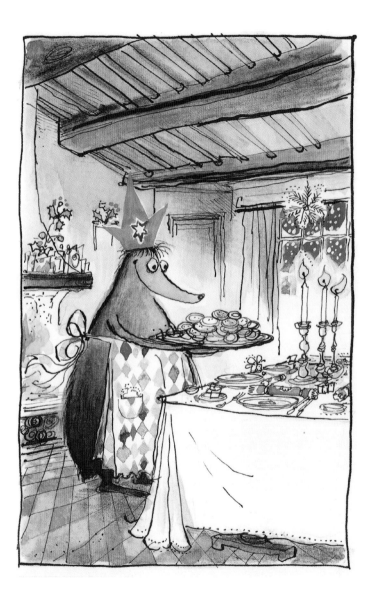

[11]

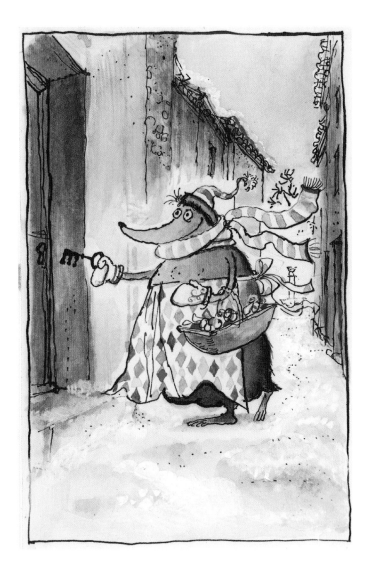

[**12**]

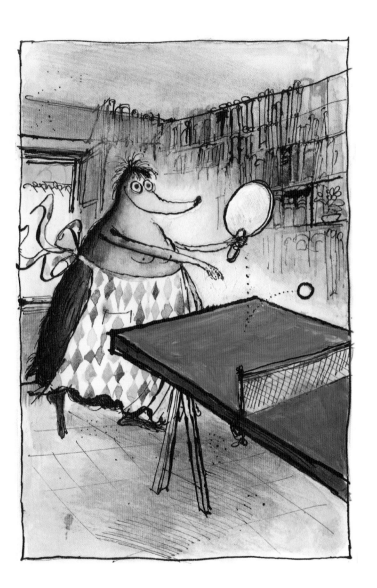

[13]

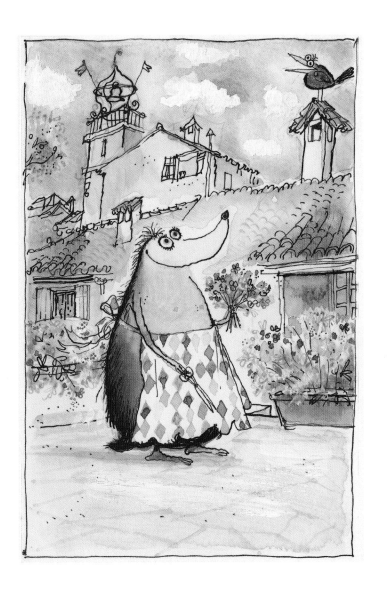

[14]

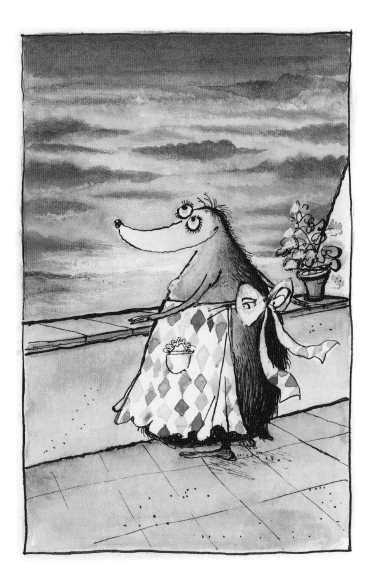

[15]

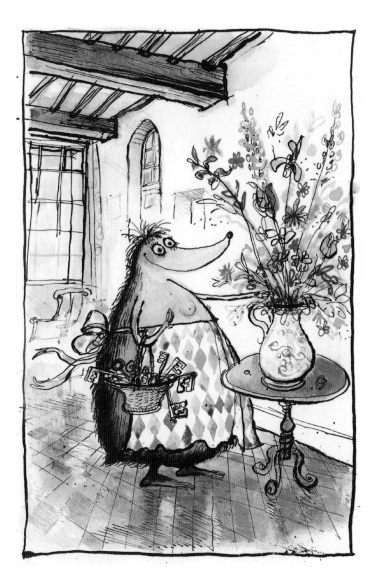

[16]

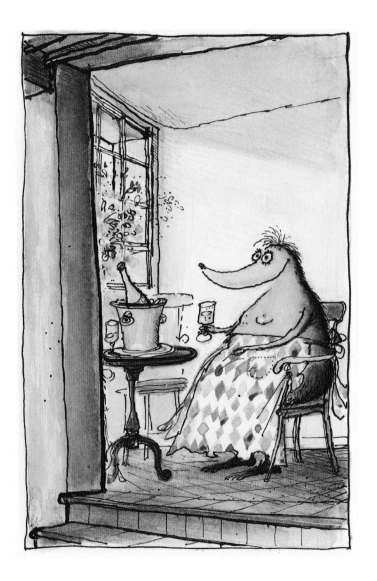

[17]

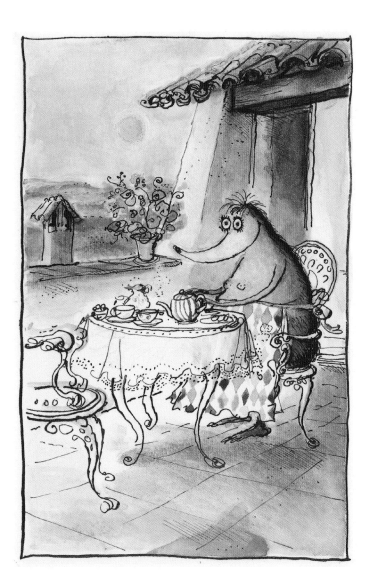

[18]

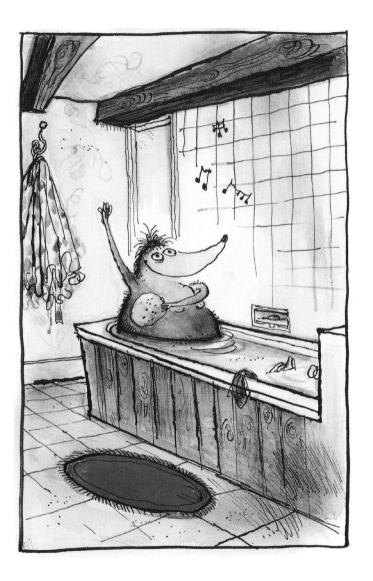

[19]

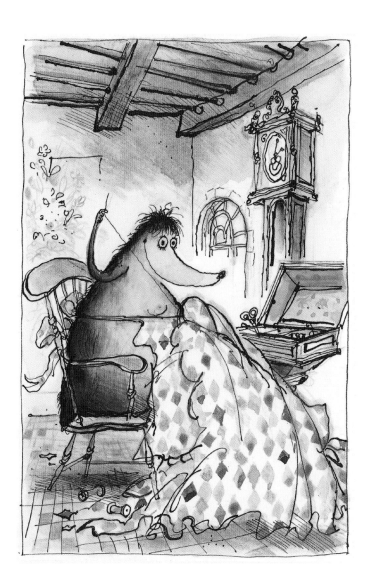

[20]

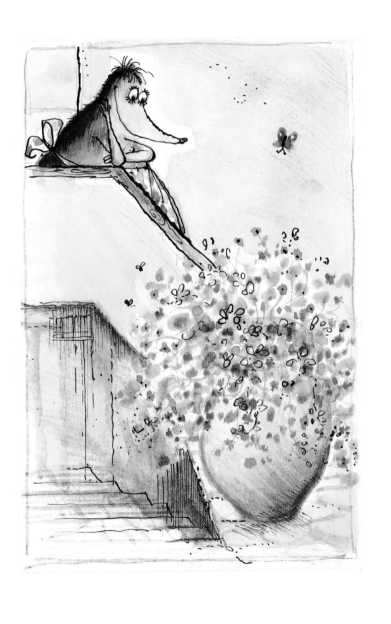

[21]

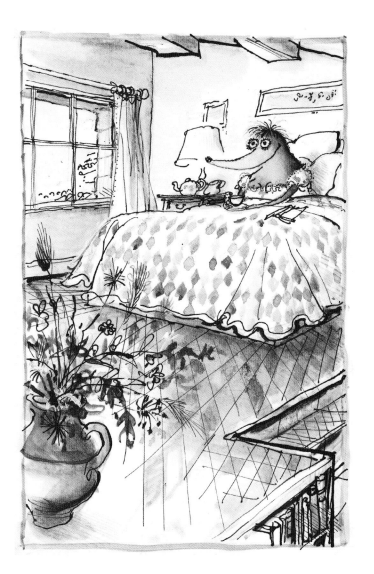

[22]

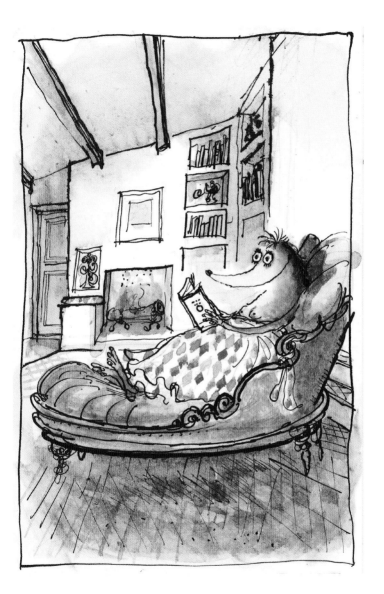

[23]

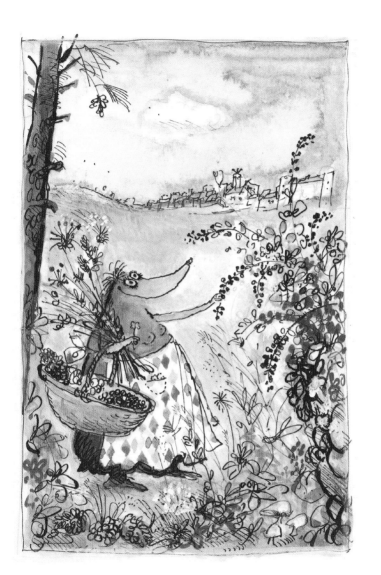

[24]

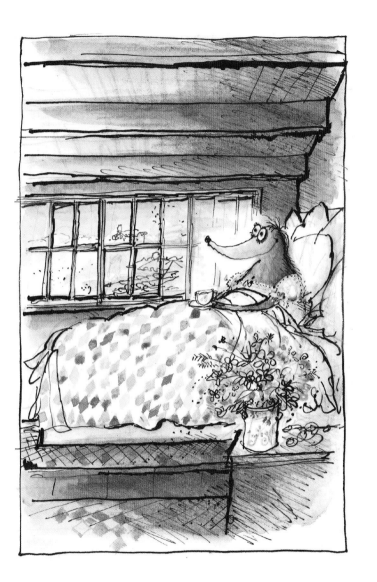

[25]

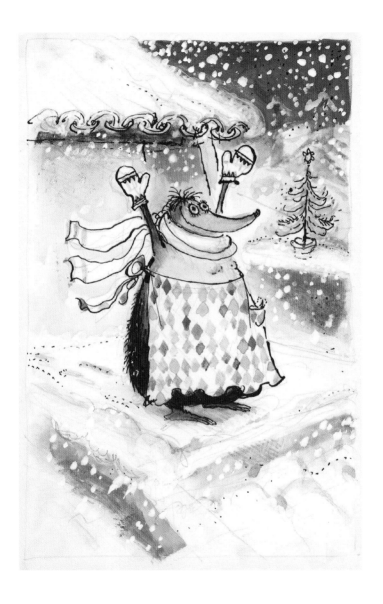

[26]

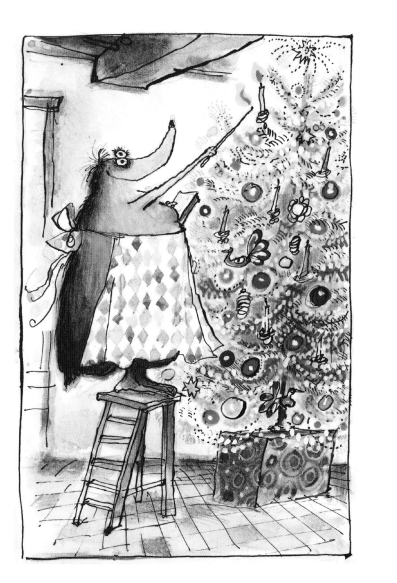

[27]

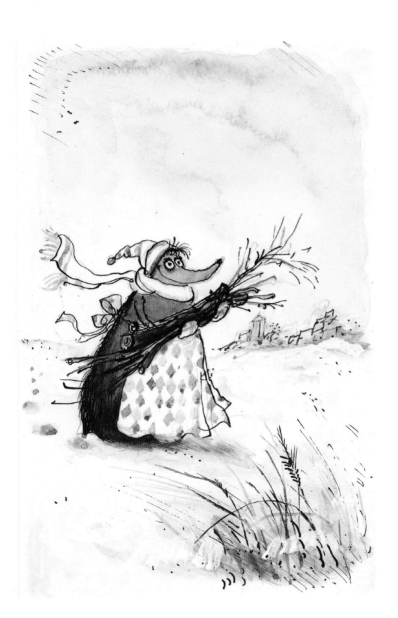

[28]

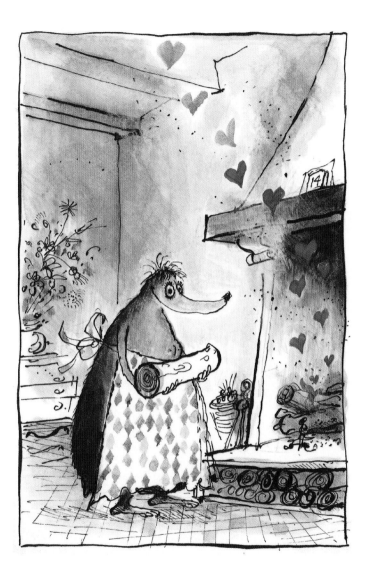

[**29**]

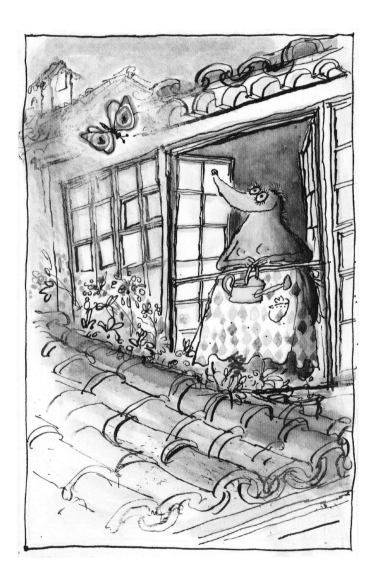

[30]

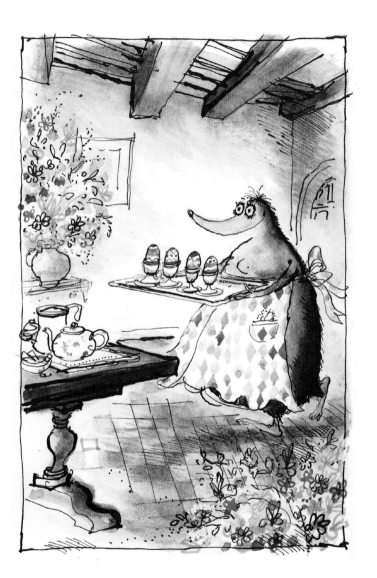

[31]

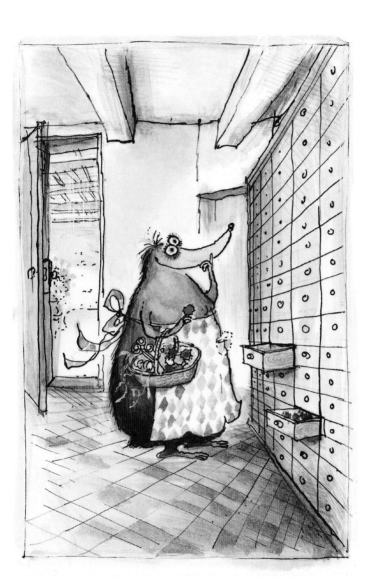

[32]

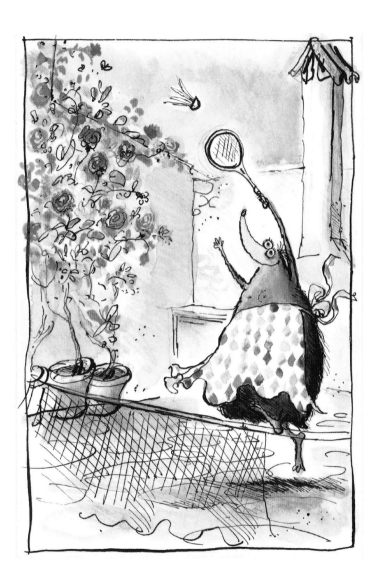

[33]

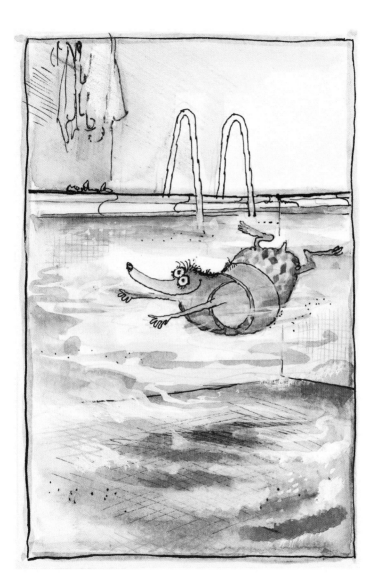

[34]

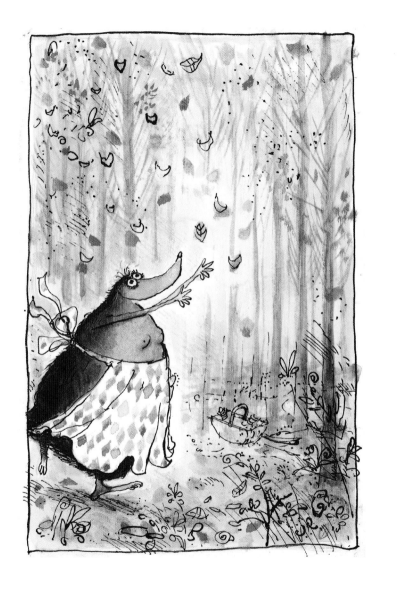

[35]

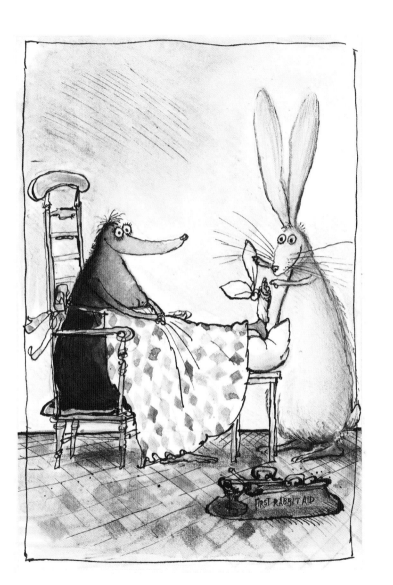

[36]

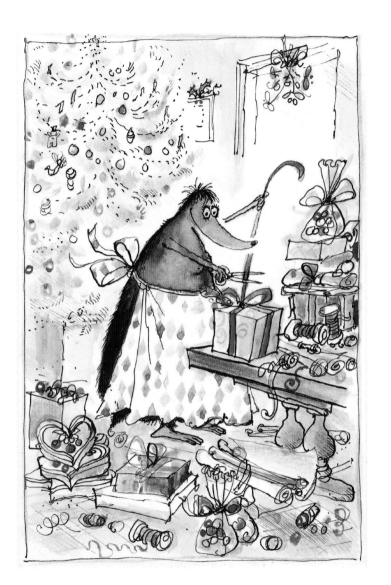

[37]

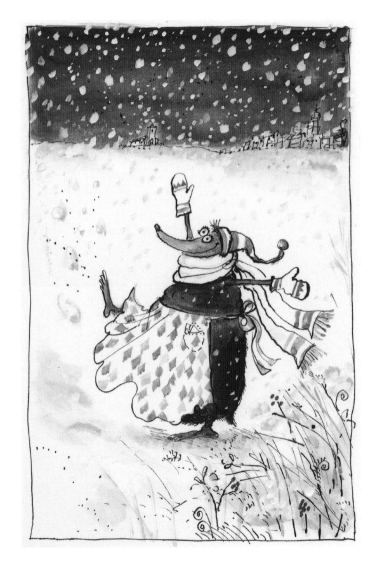

[38]

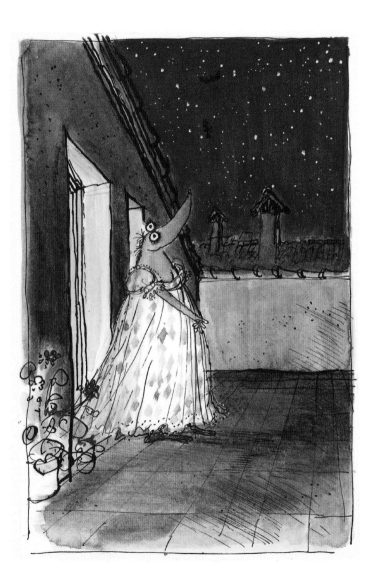

[39]

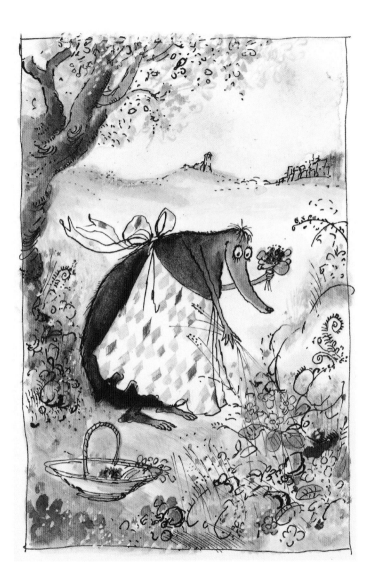

[40]

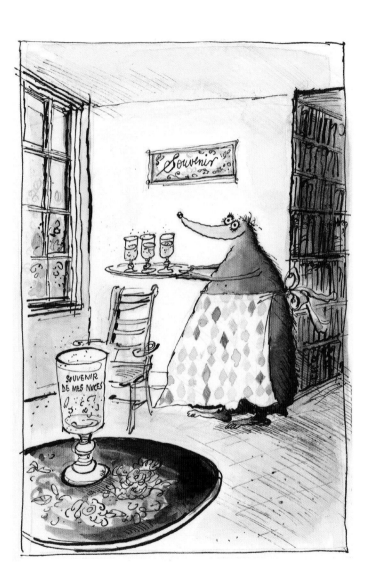

[41]

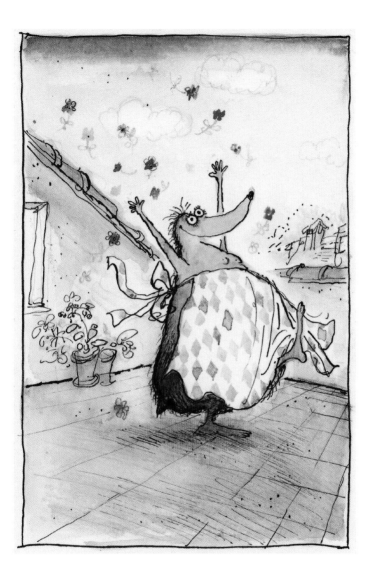

[42]

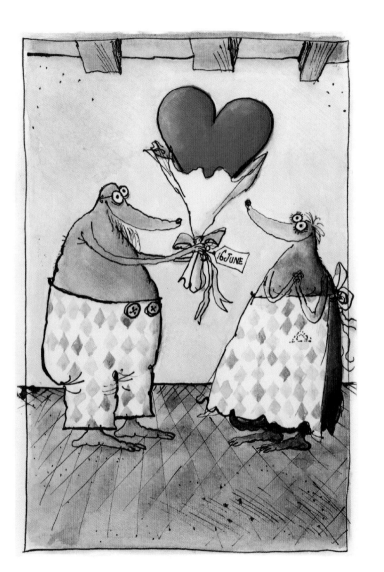

[43]

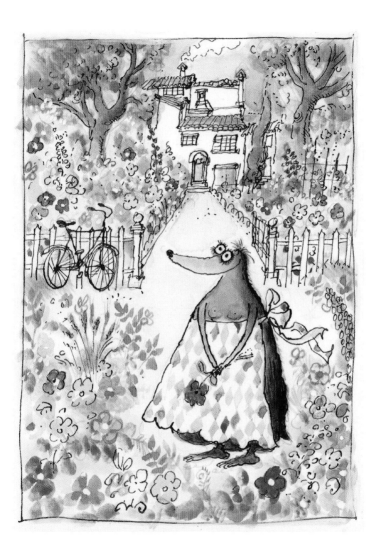

[44]

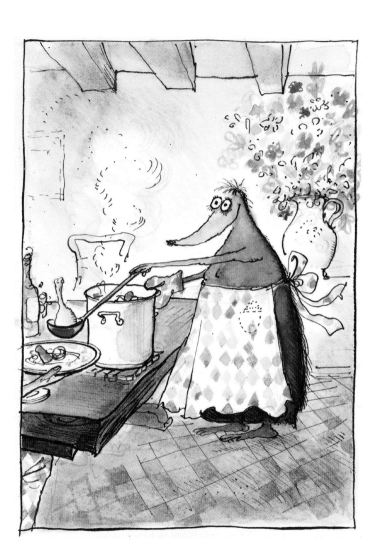

[45]

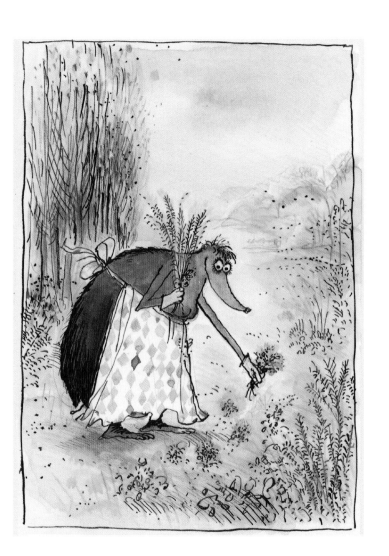

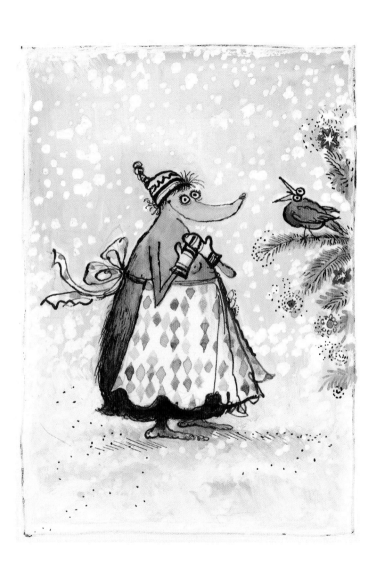

[47]

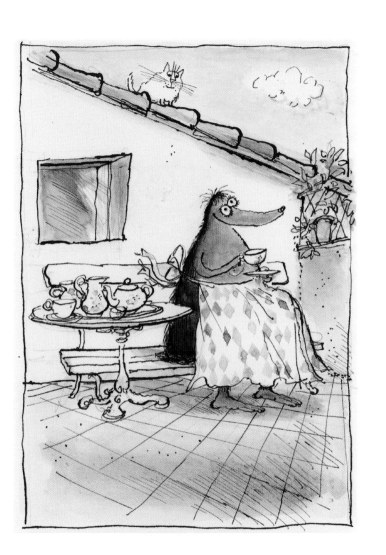

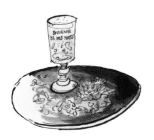

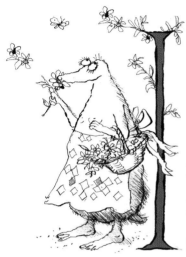

In September 1969 Ronald and I bought a decrepit house in the south of France and he asked me to convert and restore it for us to live in.

As he has mentioned in his preface, our lives changed radically from the 31st December three months later.

Today, chemotherapy is still approached with some apprehension by all those who have to undergo it. Forty years ago, however, it was horrendous. Treatments took place every two weeks. I decided instantly that I would have bi-weekly cancer: one week prostrate, one week healthy, firmly banishing any negative feelings while I worked on the plans for the house.

Professor Léon Schwarzenberg, who saved my life (after I had been turned down by an eminent cancer specialist with the advice "Put her somewhere comfortable and help her to die as peacefully as possible"), had to work experimentally as my body refused most of the chemo ingredients in use at that time. This made everything more difficult, but life continued optimistically, thanks to Ronald.

He was wonderful throughout – a tower of strength and a continual source of pleasure. From the start he had the idea of giving me a little drawing for each chemo session and I would lie in bed, living the life he created in the pictures.

The house provided plenty of surprises to keep me busy changing and adjusting the plans. Among these was the discovery of *two* big, forgotten, buried cellars; also quite a large room with no door or windows, which appeared when part of the roof was removed to build a terrace.

The pictures in this book are reproduced in the order in which they were given to me. They record Mrs. Mole's daily life, including: the finding of the cellars – the first with imaginary gold coins to sweep up, the second converted into a swimming-pool; the installation of a bathroom; champagne or coffee moments; badminton on the terrace; table-tennis in the library; the celebration of Christmas; an injured toe; romantic reflections by moonlight; etc.; etc. It was wonderful!

Every time he came to give me another treatment, Léon's first question would be: "Where's the new drawing?"

The sessions continued for five years and the house gradually turned into our present home in which we have been able to continue our happy life together – all thanks to Ronald and, of course, Mrs. Mole.

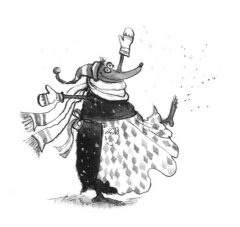

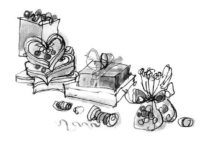

Blue Door
An imprint of HarperCollins*Publishers*
77–85 Fulham Palace Road,
Hammersmith, London W6 8JB

www.harpercollins.co.uk

First published as a special limited edition of 196 copies
by Artists' Choice Editions

This edition published by Blue Door in 2011
1

Copyright © Ronald Searle 2010

The original artwork forms part of the Searle archive in the Deutsches Museum
für Karikatur und Zeichenkunst: Wilhelm Busch, Hannover

A catalogue record of this book is
available from the British Library

ISBN 978-0-00-744910-1

Printed and bound in Italy by L.E.G.O. SpA